KT-526-433

An Introduction to Coping with

Insomnia and Sleep Problems

2nd Edition

Colin A. Espie

ROBINSON

ROBINSON

First published in Great Britain in 2011 by Robinson
an imprint of Constable & Robinson Ltd

This edition published in 2017 by Robinson

1 3 5 7 9 10 8 6 4 2

A CIP catalogue record for this book
is available from the British Library.

Important note
This book is not intended as a substitute for medical advice
or treatment. Any person with a condition requiring medical
attention should consult a qualified medical practitioner
or suitable therapist.

ISBN: 978-1-47213-854-5

Typeset in Bembo by Initial Typesetting Services, Edinburgh
Printed and bound in Great Britain by
CPI Group (UK) Ltd, Croydon CR0 4YY

Papers used by Robinson are from well-managed forests
and other responsible sources.

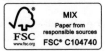

Robinson
An imprint of
Little, Brown Book Group
Carmelite House
50 Victoria Embankment
London EC4Y 0DZ

An Hachette UK Company
www.hachette.co.uk

www.littlebrown.co.uk

Contents

About This Book

Everyone has the occasional night of poor sleep, and most of us have had times when we've found it hard to get to sleep or stay asleep when we're stressed or worried about something. Usually these problems go away quite quickly and normal sleep returns. However, sleeping problems can also become more constant, and this is when the term 'insomnia' is commonly used.

The first part of this book sets out to help you understand what insomnia is, and also to find out about some other less-well-known sleep disorders in case they may be playing a part in your difficulties. The second part will show you some methods that you can use to help get your sleep back on track. All of the methods included in this booklet are evidence based. This means that they've all been tested in clinical trials and shown to help, if people stick at using them. This point must be stressed because, once you have persistent insomnia (when you rarely, or never, get a good night's sleep), it can be difficult to overcome it unless you're prepared to make some changes in the way you behave and changes in the way you think about sleep.

You may well find that following this book will be enough to sort out your sleep problems. It would be best to follow the book carefully, as a short course in fixing your sleep pattern. You'll see that it is often helpful to write things down, and the book gives you some tools to use that will help you with this. It's also useful to read parts over again, perhaps several times. Some simple things can help many people change their routines and their way of thinking to help them sleep better.

This book is based on Cognitive Behavioural Therapy (CBT), which is a practical, down-to-earth approach which has a successful record in helping people with problems to transform their lives through changing the way they think and act. Of course, there's only a limited amount of material that can be provided in such a short book, so don't be too put off if you don't get the results you're hoping for. There are more detailed books about Cognitive Behavioural Therapy for insomnia available. Also, if you don't make as much progress as you would wish, then you should talk to your GP about your sleeping problems. This is particularly important if you think that you may have a sleep disorder other than insomnia.

Good luck with improving your sleep!

Professor Colin A. Espie

Part 1: ABOUT INSOMNIA

1

What is Insomnia?

Insomnia: what it means

You probably know all too well what insomnia is! It's a miserable experience when you don't sleep well at night, and having poor sleep affects how you feel during the day. So perhaps you don't really need me to tell you!

But then again, maybe it's useful to confirm whether or not you have a clinical problem with your sleep. Here's a checklist of what insomnia is. By working through this list, you'll be able to sum up the nature of your night-time sleep disturbance, its effects on your day-to-day life and, overall, how bad your problem is. You'll also be able to see what type of insomnia disorder you're suffering from.

To help you, the example shown in Figure 1 (overleaf) is of a mild but persistent sleep-maintenance insomnia with daytime effects of fatigue and mood disturbance (which means that the person has had

Night-time (My problem is that...)	Check (→)	
I can't get to sleep at the start of the night	→	Sleep-onset Insomnia
I can't stay asleep during the night	→	Sleep-maintenance Insomnia
I can't get to sleep AND I can't stay asleep	→	Mixed Insomnia
Daytime (My poor sleep results in...)	Check (→)	
Fatigue or low energy	→	
Daytime sleepiness	→	
Mental impairments (e.g. attention, memory)	→	Insomnia with daytime consequences
Mood disturbance (e.g. irritability, feeling low)	→	
Poor performance (e.g. work, responsibilities)	→	
Problems with others (e.g. family, friends)	→	
Severity (These are problems for me...)	Check (→)	
Once or twice a week	→	Mild
Three or more nights a week	→	Severe
For less than three months	→	Acute
For more than three months	→	Persistent

FIGURE 1

Night-time (My problem is that...)	Check (→)	
I can't get to sleep at the start of the night	→	Sleep-onset Insomnia
I can't stay asleep during the night	→	Sleep-maintenance Insomnia
I can't get to sleep AND I can't stay asleep	→	Mixed Insomnia
Daytime (My poor sleep results in...)	Check (→)	
Fatigue or low energy	→	
Daytime sleepiness	→	
Mental impairments (e.g. attention, memory)	→	Insomnia with daytime consequences
Mood disturbance (e.g. irritability, feeling low)	→	
Poor performance (e.g. work, responsibilities)	→	
Problems with others (e.g. family, friends)	→	
Severity (These are problems for me...)	Check (→)	
Once or twice a week	→	Mild
Three or more nights a week	→	Severe
For less than three months	→	Acute
For more than three months	→	Persistent

FIGURE 2

trouble sleeping one or two nights a week for several months, and so feels tired and moody during the day).

Fill out Figure 2 (page 5) to find out your kind of sleep problem, and then write down your experience below.

_____

_____

_____

_____

_____

_____

Now, whatever type of insomnia you may have, try to remember this, as it's quite important: insomnia is really a 24-hour disorder – it's not just about difficulty sleeping at night. It's also a daytime problem and, in fact, this is what drives many people to seek help. People can just about put up with not sleeping, but when they're irritable or tired during the day, and perhaps not coping with work or relationships, as well as not sleeping, then that's quite a different matter.

Other disorders of sleep

So far so good. The next thing is to check to see if you might have any other forms of sleep disorder. Different types of sleep problems can go together, or we may think that we have one type when in fact we have another.

So here's another checklist! In each set of questions in the table on pages 9–11, you'll see that there's a lead question in bold, and if you answer 'yes' to that, you should then go on and look at the questions just beneath it. Do the same for each set of questions.

You can use Figure 3 as a kind of screening tool in case you may have difficulty with narcolepsy (which is a disorder of excessive daytime sleepiness), obstructive sleep apnoea (a sleep-related breathing disorder that also makes us really sleepy), or a sleep motor disorder (like periodic limb movement disorder or restless legs syndrome). There are also sections in Figure 3 on what we call parasomnias and circadian rhythm sleep disorders. Here's a brief word on each of these.

Parasomnias are divided into those sleep problems that happen during dreaming rapid-eye-movement (REM) sleep, such as nightmares, and those problems that occur during non-REM sleep (such as sleepwalking and night terrors). Circadian rhythm sleep disorders happen when the body-clock is out of sync with the clock on the wall. Common examples of these, which tend to be short lived, include jet lag and problems caused by shift work. In other words, the problem sorts itself out naturally over time. But there are some disorders of the body-clock that can be more long-lasting.

If you answered 'yes' to any of the five areas in Figure 2, you may wish to see your GP for further advice.

If you want to have another assessment of your sleep you can fill out the 'Great British Sleep Survey' at www.greatbritishsleepsurvey.com. After you fill out the questions, the website will give you a report on your sleep. The survey is provided by Sleepio, an organisation trying to find new ways to help people sleep better.

FIGURE 3

---

1. Narcolepsy

a. **Do you sometimes fall asleep in the daytime completely without warning?**
b. Is it impossible to resist 'sleep attacks' during the day?
c. Do you collapse or have extreme muscle weakness triggered by extreme emotion?
d. Do you have visual hallucinations, either just as you fall asleep or when you wake in the morning?
e. Are you paralysed and unable to move when you wake up from your sleep?

(If the answer to question 1a is 'yes', and the answer to questions 1b or 1c or 1d or 1e is also 'yes', this might mean possible narcolepsy.)

2. Sleep breathing disorder

a. **Are you a very heavy snorer?**
b. Does your partner say that you sometimes stop breathing when you are asleep?
c. Do you often wake up gasping for breath?
d. Are you often very sleepy during the day or do you fall asleep without wanting to?

(If the answer to question 1a is 'yes', and the answer to questions 1b or 1c or 1d is also 'yes', this might mean possible sleep breathing disorder.)

3. Periodic Limb Movement Syndrome (PLMS)/Restless Legs Syndrome (RLS)

a. **Do your legs often twitch or jerk or can you not keep still in bed?**

b. Is it very difficult to get to sleep because of repeated muscle jerks?

c. Do you frequently wake from sleep with sudden jerky movements or with a compulsion to move your legs?

d. Do you simply have to get out of bed and pace around to get rid of these feelings?

(If the answer to question 1a is 'yes', and the answer to questions 1b or 1c or 1d is also 'yes', this might mean possible PLMS/RLS.)

4. Circadian Rhythm Sleep Disorder (CRSD)

a. **Do you tend to sleep well but just at the 'wrong times'?**

b. Can you sleep well enough, but only if you stay up very late?

c. Are you in a very sound sleep at normal waking time and able to sleep on for hours more?

d. Can you sleep well enough, but only if you go to bed very early?

e. Do you wake very early, bright and alert and no longer sleepy?

(If the answer to question 1a is 'yes', and the answer
to questions 1b or 1c or 1d or 1e is also 'yes', this
might mean possible CRSD.)

5. Parasomnia

a. **Are there unusual behaviours associated
with your sleep that trouble you or that
are dangerous?**
b. Do you sleepwalk frequently and run the risk
of injuring yourself or others?
c. Do you often have night terrors when you are
extremely distressed but not properly awake?
d. Do you act out your dreams and risk injuring
yourself or others?
e. Do you have terrible recurring nightmares?

(If the answer to question 1a is 'yes', and the answer
to questions 1b or 1c or 1d or 1e is also 'yes', this
might mean possible parasomnia.)

Sleep and mood

We've looked at the possibility that you have an
insomnia disorder, and the possibility that you could
have some other type of sleep problem instead of,
or as well as, insomnia. Before moving on, though,
let's look more closely at the relationship between
our sleep and our mood.

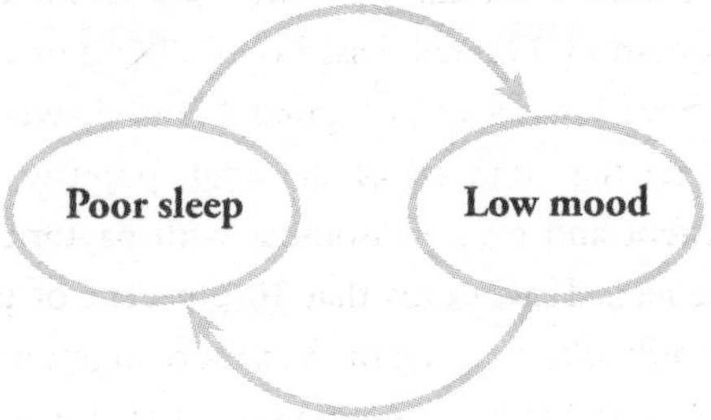

FIGURE 4

Often when people have a problem sleeping, they also have a problem with how they feel emotionally. Most commonly, this could be in the form of feeling worried/anxious or down/depressed. As you can see in Figure 4, this is pretty much a two-way street! If we become more emotionally upset, then our sleep is likely to get worse, but it also works the other way round: if our sleep gets worse, then we are more likely to become emotionally upset. In fact, having a long-term problem with insomnia is now known to make it more likely that you could develop depression. So it is certainly worth doing something about an insomnia problem!

How common is insomnia?

Before looking at what causes insomnia, it is important to pause to think about just how common it is.

There have been many research studies looking at this question. Overall, based on the kind of criteria you have looked at in Figures 1 and 2, we could estimate that 1 in 10 of the adult population has persistent and severe insomnia with daytime consequences. This means that 10 per cent of people have difficulty sleeping on 3 or more nights a week, that this problem has gone on for at least 3 months, and it is causing them problems such as tiredness and moodiness during the day. In adults over the age of 65, the number of people with persistent and severe insomnia could be as high as 1 in 5.

About 15 years ago, the largest ever survey of the mental health of the UK population was conducted. The graph on page 15 (Figure 5) is taken from that survey and reveals just how common sleep problems are. In this case, the questions for each symptom are not very precise, so you get higher rates for insomnia (more like 30 per cent). The graph shows that, for both men and women, sleep problems, tiredness and irritability are by far the most common symptoms of mental distress that people experience. Sleep problems are much more common than worry, depression and anxiety.

So, you can feel reassured that you are in good company! There are plenty of us who could do with some help with our insomnia.

Figure 5 (see opposite)
Insomnia is a common problem
affecting a third of adults.

(Reproduced by permission of Her Majesty's Stationery Office from
N. Singleton, R. Bumpstead, M. O'Brien, A. Lee & H. Meltzer
Kales, 'Psychiatric Morbidity among Adults Living in Private House-
holds'. The Office for National Statistics, HMSO, 2001.)

FIGURE 5

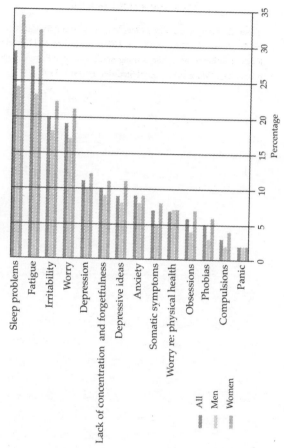

2

What Causes Insomnia?

This is one of the most common questions asked about insomnia. There are different answers for every individual person's problem, but there are also some common factors. Let me explain.

Predisposing, precipitating and perpetuating factors

One of the best ways to think about how insomnia develops is to consider the three Ps.

The first P refers to predisposing factors. This means the types of things that can make it more likely that you will develop insomnia, compared to somebody else. Perhaps your family has a history of poor sleep, perhaps you're the type of person who tends to react to stress or is generally very anxious, or perhaps you've had a lot of upheavals at home or at work. These are all things that might make you more likely to have poor sleep. But predisposing factors in themselves aren't enough to cause insomnia.

The second P stands for precipitating or triggering factors. This means events that affect you and stop you sleeping well. You might have been under quite a bit of stress because of a particular reason, such as an illness, or bereavement, or a period of unemployment. This might mean that you develop acute insomnia (acute insomnia is when you have sleeping problems for less than 3 months). Precipitating factors, however, can also be more everyday things, like noises from outside disturbing your sleep, or changes in the house, like having a new baby. So please note that precipitating factors are not always bad. Any major changes – good or bad – can cause stress and lead to acute insomnia.

FIGURE 6

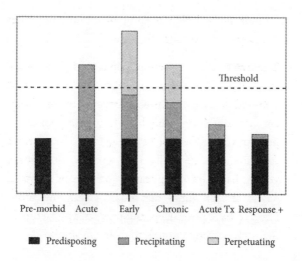

The third P stands for perpetuating factors meaning the things that keep a sleep problem going once it's started. Most commonly, people say that they remember when their sleep problem started, but they don't understand what's kept it going for so long! This is exactly what is meant by perpetuation – for some reason, the problem remains, keeping the sleep problem above that troublesome threshold (Figure 6) until effective treatment comes along.

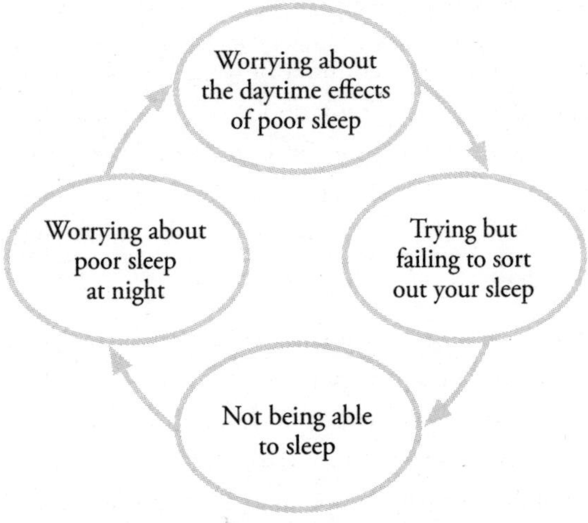

Worrying about
the daytime effects
of poor sleep

Worrying about
poor sleep
at night

Trying but
failing to sort
out your sleep

Not being able
to sleep

FIGURE 7

The most common problem that people have is a vicious cycle of not being able to sleep, becoming concerned and worried about not sleeping, and about the daytime effects of not sleeping well at night, and trying unsuccessfully to fix things, leading to a continued inability to sleep. This cycle leads to a lot of frustration and anxiety, and of course makes the insomnia worse, not better. This is when persistent insomnia (when it lasts more than 3 months) really takes hold!

A good-enough explanation

Now it is time to consider how your problem may have developed. Think about why you may have been likely to develop insomnia in the first place, what the triggering factors were and, most importantly, what is keeping it going now. Think about the vicious cycle – does that make sense to you?

It can be very helpful to write down your own story, just in a paragraph or two. You can keep it private. Many people find doing this helpful in order to give themselves what can be called 'a good-enough explanation' for their sleep problem. This is something you can refer to again and again, and it can help you move on to sort out the problem. But be warned, most people never achieve a total explanation so just try to make it a 'good-enough explanation'. Don't spend too much time trying to make the explanation perfect. In the end, it is effective action, not just thinking about your problem, which will make a difference to your sleep.

3

Different Treatments for Insomnia

No doubt you've already been trying your best to overcome your insomnia. There are three approaches that people often try – two of them (medication and psychological therapies) have at some level been shown to be effective, while there is currently no scientific evidence that the third approach (other therapies) works.

Medication

'Taking something' to help us sleep is an ancient tradition. Even in the distant past people took pills or potions to help them sleep. Nowadays, there are a variety of sleeping pills. These include drugs known as benzodiazepines (often with a name ending with -epam), and a similar group (often beginning with the letter z) which are a bit less habit-forming, though they act in the same way. Pills can help people get to sleep, but they may not work in the long term. Consequently, UK and international health guidelines recommend sleeping pills only for the short term (a few days or weeks at most), or for occasional use. Sleeping pills are not suitable for people with a persistent insomnia problem that has lasted many months or years.

Sometimes people are given medications that are meant for another purpose but, as a side-effect, cause drowsiness. These drugs might be anti-depressant drugs (intended for people who are depressed) or anti-histamine drugs (for allergies such as hay fever). This is known as 'off-label prescribing'. Doctors are allowed to do this, but there is little scientific evidence to show that these medicines are effective in treating insomnia. Some doctors prefer these kinds of drugs because they can prescribe them for a longer length of time than sleeping pills.

Finally, there is melatonin. This is a natural hormone that the brain produces in the late evening and throughout the night. Some studies suggest that tablets containing melatonin taken several hours before bedtime can help people get to sleep more quickly. However, we can't be sure that they will work in the long term, so melatonin is not the right answer for persistent insomnia. Some people prefer the idea of a 'natural' product over a sleeping pill but as with sleeping pills, if you stop taking melatonin, you can go back to your old sleeping problems almost immediately.

Psychological therapies

There's a lot of evidence that psychological treatments for insomnia, based mostly on Cognitive Behavioural Therapy (CBT) techniques, work in the long term as well as the short term. This is because it's often our thoughts, behaviour and emotions which stop us from sleeping. Psychological therapies deal with these thoughts, behaviour and emotions, and so prevent the vicious cycle that we looked at in the last chapter.

This book introduces some of the CBT methods that have been the most helpful for people with sleep problems. You can find out how to get more information on CBT by looking at the 'Other Things that Might Help' section at the back of this book. During the past 25 years, over 150 clinical trials of CBT in the treatment of insomnia have been conducted, showing that 70 per cent of people gain lasting benefit.

Another development that has some scientific support is the use of bright light. The cycle of when we sleep and when we wake is regulated by natural light. Exposure to natural light and to artificial bright light (using a 'light-box') can help us to control our phases of sleep. However, the evidence suggests that using bright light is best for the treatment of circadian rhythm sleep disorders rather than insomnia. Bright light can be used along with CBT as part of a treatment programme for insomnia, but it only seems to work when someone has great difficulty getting to sleep every night, or wakes up very early every morning.

Other therapies

Some people believe in the benefits of things like camomile tea, warm milky drinks, special pillows, herbal remedies, homeopathic medicines, neuro-linguistic programming, binaural beats and so on. However, there is no research evidence to support the benefits of any of these as a treatment for insomnia. Indeed, many people list these therapies as the things they have already tried unsuccessfully. There is also an enormous range of remedies available in pharmacies, but be aware that we don't know how effective they really are.

Part 2: COPING WITH INSOMNIA

4

Setting Clear Goals

Personal goals

Before you set out on a journey, it's always a good idea to know what your destination is! Once you know that, then you can plan ahead. Now, you are probably thinking that your destination's fairly obvious – you can't sleep and you just want to be able to sleep again. But it's important to develop a specific and clear personal goal.

Look back to the beginning of this book where you thought about the type of insomnia you have, and also about the way your poor sleep affects your day-to-day life. Most likely, your personal goal will be pretty much the opposite of what you have been experiencing. For example, if your problem is that you wake up at night, and this affects your mood and your relationships, then your goal might be something like, 'I want to be able to sleep right through, be in a better frame of mind during the daytime, and be able to get on better with other people.' Below, write down what you think would be the best statement to summarise your goal. Try to use your own words.

_____

_____

_____

_____

_____

_____

_____

Keeping a sleep diary

Now that you have set your goal, it's useful to think about how you can measure your sleep. A sleep diary is a tool you can use to track your progress. See overleaf for an example of what this should look like (Figure 8). Fill in a column each morning soon after you wake up, and over time this will give you a record of how well you are sleeping. If you compare the goal that you wrote in the box to the questions listed down the side of the diary, you will see that some questions are more relevant to you than others. For example, if you mainly have a problem getting to sleep, then question 6 will be very important. Your answers to the questions that are most relevant to your goal will help you see how you are getting on. Also, make sure you answer questions 11 and 12, as they will help to give you a good overall idea of how you are doing. Keep on filling out the diary every day until you feel that you have overcome your long-term sleep problem.

FIGURE 7

MEASURING THE PATTERN OF YOUR SLEEP	DAY 1	DAY 2	DAY 3	DAY 4	DAY 5	DAY 6	DAY 7
1. Did you nap at any point yesterday? If yes, for how long (minutes)?							
2. What time did you finally wake up this morning?							
3. At what time did you rise from bed this morning?							
4. At what time did you go to bed last night?							
5. At what time did you switch off the light intending to go to sleep?							
6. How long did it take you to fall asleep (minutes)?							
7. How long were you awake during the night because of these awakenings (total minutes)?							

8. About how long did you sleep altogether (hours/minutes)?							
9. How much alcohol did you have last night?							
10. Did you take sleeping pills to help you sleep last night? If so, how many?							

MEASURING THE QUALITY OF YOUR SLEEP

11. How refreshed do you feel this morning? 0 1 2 3 4 not at all moderately very							
12. How would you rate the overall quality of your sleep last night? 0 1 2 3 4 poor very good							

Sleep efficiency

Now think about an extra goal, one that you may never have heard about before. This goal is to increase your sleep efficiency. People with insomnia are inefficient sleepers. That is, they only sleep for part of the night, whereas good sleepers sleep for most of it. Look at the examples opposite.

Most good sleepers manage around 90 per cent sleep efficiency – and that's pretty good! This would be the equivalent of spending 8 hours in bed (480 minutes), and only having a total of 48 minutes (10 per cent) throughout that whole time awake. Take a moment now to work out your own sleep efficiency by putting some figures into the equation opposite (Figure 9) and calculating your score.

> Sarah goes to bed at 11 p.m. and gets up at 7 a.m. She sleeps all of the 8 hours between these times. This means that Sarah is a very efficient sleeper indeed – in fact she has 100 per cent sleep efficiency because she sleeps absolutely all of the time she spends in bed.

John also goes to bed at 11 p.m. and gets up at 7 a.m. He takes 45 minutes to fall asleep and is awake during the night for another 90 minutes. This means that John is awake for 2 hours 15 minutes. He sleeps for 5 hours 45 minutes of the 8 hours that he is in bed. John's sleep efficiency therefore is only 72 per cent.

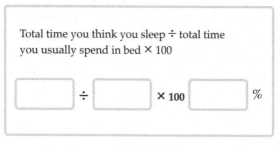

Total time you think you sleep ÷ total time you usually spend in bed × 100

$$\boxed{} \div \boxed{} \times 100 \boxed{} \%$$

Figure 9

OK, now compare your sleep efficiency (%) with the chart in Figure 10. You should be able to see how far below 90 per cent your sleep efficiency is, and also what kind of 'banding' of sleep quality it relates to. Your additional goal then is to get your sleep efficiency up to 90 per cent. Why not write this alongside where you wrote your goal on page 28.

Total sleep time (hours)

Time in bed (hours) \ Hours	3	3.5	4	4.5	5	5.5	6	6.5	7	7.5	8	8.5	9	9.5	10
3	100														
3.5	86	100													
4	75	88	100												
4.5	67	78	89	100											
5	60	70	80	90	100										
5.5	55	64	73	82	91	100									
6	50	58	67	75	83	92	100								
6.5	45	54	62	69	77	85	92	100							
7	43	50	57	64	71	79	86	93	100						
7.5	40	47	53	60	67	73	80	87	93	100					
8	37	44	50	56	63	69	75	81	88	94	100				
8.5	35	41	47	53	59	65	71	76	82	88	94	100			
9	33	39	44	50	56	61	67	72	78	83	89	94	100		
9.5	32	37	42	47	53	58	63	68	74	79	84	89	95	100	
10	30	35	40	45	50	55	60	65	70	75	80	85	90	95	100

FIGURE 10 Sleep Efficiency (%)

5

Improving Your Sleep Hygiene

What is sleep hygiene?

Sleep hygiene is quite an odd phrase because it has got nothing really to do with hygiene. It's a list of the things you can control in order to make a good night's sleep more likely.

However, sleep hygiene instructions on their own aren't really effective for treating persistent insomnia, and having a list of dos and don'ts doesn't usually help us to change the way we act. For example, someone who is overweight might be advised to eat more fruit and vegetables, eat fewer carbohydrates and take more exercise, but that does not really give them any tools to help them. If you have tried sleep hygiene and it hasn't really worked, do not become demoralised, because Cognitive Behavioural Therapy offers many other ways to help you.

If you want to 'refresh' on your sleep hygiene, use the instruction in Figure 11 to help you overcome your sleep problem.

Lifestyle factors

As you can see from Figure 11, there are lifestyle factors and bedroom factors associated with good sleep hygiene. For example, it's best not to drink caffeinated (tea/coffee) or alcoholic drinks, or to have a main meal, within 4 hours of going to bed. A small snack at supper time shouldn't be a problem. Likewise, although exercise is good for our physical and mental health, it's best not to exercise within 2 hours of going to bed because it tends to keep us awake. Smoking, of course, is bad for our health but, if you must smoke, then you should cut down before bedtime and try not to smoke during the night. Not only is nicotine a stimulant drug (like caffeine), your body may also wake you up craving a cigarette.

Lifestyle Factors

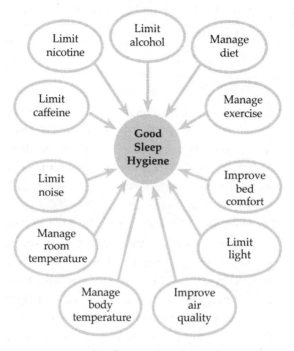

Bedroom Factors

FIGURE 11

Bedroom factors

The bedroom factors in Figure 11 are also important. Most of these factors concern making the bedroom suitable for sleep, that is, limiting noise (but that does not mean that you need complete silence), making it dark (but not necessarily pitch black), and making sure that you have a comfortable mattress and pillows. Temperature is important. The ideal room temperature is around 18°C (64°F) – not too hot and not too cold. If anything, sleep prefers the cool, so you shouldn't be too warm in bed. A hot bath immediately before going to bed is likely to keep us awake.

Good sleep hygiene gives us a starting point so that we can improve our approach to sleep, but don't be surprised if this isn't enough on its own.

Improving Your Preparation for Sleep

Bedtime wind-down

You shouldn't expect just to fall into bed and go to sleep because you happen to think it's 'bedtime'. There are a few people who can do that, but as you have a sleep problem it's likely your preparation for sleep could almost certainly be better.

Developing a wind-down routine, starting at least 60–90 minutes before bed, so that you can begin relaxing and preparing for sleep, will help you fall asleep once you are in bed.

Your routine could include things like slowing down your work/activity and then stopping it, and having some relaxation time before you start getting ready for bed. Figure 12 shows a good wind-down routine, but it's important for you to work out your own routine which suits your own interests and timelines. Bear in mind that your routine should be carefully planned, but make sure also that it is not too strict, or you may become anxious or

disappointed if you cannot do everything on time.
The point is to help you relax, not to get stressed.

Approximate time	Planned schedule
7.30	Put day to rest using 'rehearsal and planning time'
7.45 – 8.30	Complete work/household activities of primary importance
8.30 – 10.00	Complete other activities
10.00 – 11.15	Work/activity completed Relaxation time (reading, TV, relaxation exercise etc.)
11.15	Pre-bed sequence (lock up, change, wash)
11.30	Retire to bed Practise relaxation

Bedtime wind-down period

FIGURE 12

The routine in Figure 12 covers around 4 hours, so
think about what you'll do throughout the whole
evening. You should pay particular attention to the
60–90 minutes before you go to bed. The important thing is to unwind during this period.

Learning to relax

Let's first think about the importance of relaxation. There are some people who simply don't value relaxation, and that's why they don't spend time on it, and may not be any good at it!

Our lives can be so full of the words *should*, *shouldn't*, *must* and *mustn't* that we don't give ourselves permission to relax! We might even feel that we shouldn't just sit and relax for a while, especially when there are 'things that need to be done'. Does any of this sound familiar? If so, you could try to learn the value of relaxing. We're simply not designed to be on the go 24 hours a day, or to treat sleep as just a break from constant activity. Now let's look at different ways to relax.

As you can see in Figure 13 below, there are different ways of getting to a relaxed state. Some people relax by active physical means such as exercise, and others become relaxed through more mental or passive (which means gentle or inactive) pastimes such as listening to music. All of these forms of relaxation are useful, and it would help you if you could think about what activities you could do in each of the four areas in Figure 13: Active, Passive, Physical and Mental. What tools do you already have in the relaxation toolbox? What skills do you still need to develop? For example, you might already like to do a crossword, which is Active and Mental relaxation, but perhaps you could also think about going for a gentle walk, which is Physical and Passive relaxation.

	Active	**Passive**
Physical	Working out at the gym	Gently strolling
Mental	Doing crossword puzzles	Listening to music

FIGURE 13

Developing a relaxed frame of mind

Having a good mix of different types of relaxation while preparing for sleep can help. Remember that being able to relax quickly is useful, so even 5 or 10 minutes here or there can be worthwhile. When it comes to sleep, you will find that some activities are more useful than others. As mentioned earlier,

you shouldn't do strenuous physical activity immediately before bed.

Some people like to make their own relaxation
recordings to help them get in the right mood to
go to sleep. Look at the 'Other Things that Might
Help' section at the back of this book if you want to
create or download your own relaxation recording.

Before we move on from the topic of relaxation,
here are some final observations on the good sleeper.

•   Good sleepers are not students of good sleep –
    they never even think about it!

•   Try to develop a relaxed frame of mind about
    your sleep.

•   When you do practise relaxation exercises,
    remember: practice makes perfect.

Have you ever asked yourself, 'How does the good
sleeper do it?' They seem to manage to fall asleep
without ever really thinking about it, so it seems
that sleep comes naturally to them, as does the relaxation necessary to get to sleep in the first place.
Likewise, if they wake up, they seem to fall asleep
again without thinking about it.

This tells us several things. Good sleepers are not
students of sleep. They just do it automatically and

naturally. Nothing more, nothing less. Far from always thinking about how best to get to sleep and stay asleep, they seem quite relaxed about it, even though sometimes even they don't sleep well. So try to have a relaxed or even detached approach to sleep and sleeplessness rather than thinking and worrying about it too much.

As you now become more relaxed in your own attitude to sleep, and more relaxed in your preparation, you might consider that you're breaking down an old habit and building a new one. This will take time and it will take practice. Are you prepared to put in that time and that practice to change your current preparation for sleep into good sleep preparation?

7

Improving Your Bed-Sleep Connection

The good sleeper also appears to associate, or connect, bed with successful sleep. Just like salt and pepper or fish and chips, it's bed and sleep. But clearly this isn't the case for someone with insomnia. If we have sleep problems, bed is associated with anxiety even before going to bed, and with wakefulness and frustration while in bed. So you can see that the good sleeper has strong, positive associations and can adapt to make a sleeping situation better. A person with insomnia has strong but negative associations and finds it hard to adapt their behaviour to make the situation better. Sleep would be helped if the bad bed-sleep connection was changed to a healthy bed-sleep connection. Well, there are four rules that will help you to have this healthy connection between sleep and bed:

Rules to strengthen the bed–sleep connection
The bed is for sleep rule
The quarter of an hour rule
The sleepy-tired rule
The saving your sleep rule

FIGURE 14

The bed is for sleep rule

Now here's one of the instructions often found in sleep hygiene, which we talked about earlier: 'Don't use your bed for anything except sleep,' meaning that activities such as watching TV, reading and talking on the telephone are out! But, actually, when applied correctly, this should be more than a simple set of don'ts; it should be a helpful, positive instruction that connects bed with sleep.

Let's look at two illustrations of getting this rule right, using reading in bed as an example.

First, you might think there's nothing wrong with reading in bed. You know plenty of people who do – and they don't have insomnia. Well, there are plenty of people who don't have a fear of dogs, so being around a dog doesn't make them anxious or stressed. But for some people the presence of a dog means fear. It's like an automatic learned reaction: as soon as they see a dog they get scared. It's the same for people with insomnia and reading in bed. For them, reading in bed is associated with wakefulness, whereas for the good sleeper it promotes sleep.

For people with insomnia, the bedroom can be associated with anxieties and stresses that aren't there for good sleepers

So, this first rule is to bar all activities (except sexual activity) from the bedroom environment in order to help you fall asleep rapidly after you get into bed.

The quarter of an hour rule

There's very strong evidence that good sleepers fall asleep within 15 minutes or so of getting into bed. Therefore, if you want to become a good sleeper, you need to train yourself to fall asleep within an approximately 15-minute opportunity. Let's call it the quarter of an hour rule. This is long enough to fall asleep at the beginning of the night or during the night.

Good sleepers fall asleep within quarter of an hour

What is meant by a quarter of an hour opportunity? Well, simply that you don't turn that opportunity into a half-hour or longer! What good is lying awake in bed, tossing and turning, and unable to sleep? All that does is strengthen the association between bed and wakefulness. Instead, this rule says that, after a quarter of an hour, you should get up, go into another room and do something different until you feel sleepy again. Then you can give yourself another quarter of an hour opportunity in bed; but if you can't get to sleep, you should get up again and repeat this as often as is necessary.

If you follow this to its logical conclusion, the quarter of an hour rule means you'll never spend any more than a quarter of an hour at a time lying awake in bed; and so it stops the bad bed–sleep connection from building up. The quarter of an hour rule will also stop you from putting too much effort into getting to sleep. Have a look at Figure 15:

The right kind of effort	The wrong kind of effort
Being motivated	Trying too hard
Following advice	Becoming more preoccupied
Sticking to the programme	Forcing sleep
Returning to the programme	Trying to win
Refusing to give up	Becoming desperate

FIGURE 15

On the one hand, you need determination that you're going to crack this problem and become a good sleeper but, on the other, you want to avoid becoming too obsessed about sleeping.

The sleepy-tired rule

You may feel that you're already an expert in sleepiness but, actually, you may be quite poor at telling the difference between tiredness and sleepiness. If you were really good at knowing when you felt sleepy, then you might be more likely to fall asleep quickly.

To be clear, you need to learn to recognise when you are what can be called sleepy-tired. The usual signs are:

- itchy eyes

- aching muscles

- an involuntary tendency to 'nod off'

- lack of energy

- yawning

This is the way you should, ideally, be feeling when you go to bed. This is how the good sleeper feels when they are resisting sleep and trying to read their book! Tiredness does not mean that sleep is inevitable. Sleepiness is a signal from our bodies that it's time to sleep.

So, you should go to bed only when you feel sleepy-tired, not simply by habit because it's 'time to go to bed'. Also, following the quarter of an hour rule, you shouldn't go back to bed again unless you feel sleepy-tired. The connection between bed and sleep will be strongest when it's glued together by sleepiness, not by wishful thinking or desperation!

The saving your sleep rule

Finally, in this section, the connection between bed and sleep is stronger if you save all your sleep for night-time. This means that you should avoid napping in the morning, in the afternoon and in the evening. This can be hard, but a nap can reduce the need for sleep at night. We've been talking about feeling sleepy-tired, so think this through. If you did feel very sleepy-tired and had a nap, the sleepy-tiredness feeling would go away, wouldn't it? The rule then is to avoid napping completely.

However, there is one exception. If you regularly feel sleepy during the day, then you may want to look again at the questions in Figure 3 near the beginning of this book. They may point to another type of sleep disorder, rather than insomnia. People with insomnia don't tend to feel excessively sleepy, and don't fall asleep while involved in activities they enjoy. If you do feel excessively sleepy and you do fall asleep while involved in activities you enjoy, you should seek advice from your doctor. And, if you are sleepy, particularly while driving or working machinery, then you must stop and rest. Having a brief 10-minute nap under these circumstances, along with a strong caffeinated drink, should allow you to complete your journey or your activities safely.

8

Making Your Sleep Pattern the Best It Can Be

Do you feel like a well-oiled machine, operating at its best? Almost certainly not, otherwise you wouldn't be reading this book. Yet that's the way we're designed to be with good, sound, deep sleep at night, which revives us, and makes us alert, good-natured and productive during the daytime.

Remember the extra goal to make your sleep as efficient as possible? The goal is to have good-quality sleep throughout the time you are in bed, and to restore your wellbeing for the daytime. One of the first questions we need to ask then is: How much sleep do you need?

How much sleep do I need?

It may come as a surprise but there are no hard and fast rules about this, any more than there would be a hard and fast rule about what height you should be, or what shoe size you should take.

You'll have heard people talking about 'getting their 8 hours', as if 8 hours is what everyone needs. This simply isn't so. You need to find out how much sleep *you* need.

Let's take another look at the sleep efficiency equation in Chapter 4. How long did you estimate your typical sleep to be? No doubt it was less than you wanted, but let's start from where you are at the moment. If you want a really accurate answer about how long you usually sleep, keep your sleep diary for ten nights, and then work out your average sleep time on this chart overleaf (Figure 16).

By dividing your total sleep over ten nights, you'll be able to work out the length of your average night's sleep. That is your first step towards making your sleep as good as it can be.

Setting a regular amount of time in bed

Your next goal is to work out a way of achieving this same amount of sleep every night. One of the problems of insomnia is the sometimes large difference in the amount of sleep you get from night to night. So, however much or little sleep you're getting, it's important to work towards getting the same amount every single night.

Night	Amount of time I slept
1	
2	
3	
4	
5	
6	
7	
8	
9	
10	

Total amount of sleep over 10 days _____

My average sleep time _____

FIGURE 16

Now, let's decide on a rising time, or getting-up time. It is best to have a set time for getting up every morning, seven nights a week, until you get your sleep problem sorted. Note that down here.

My getting-up time will be —————

The next thing is to set a threshold time for going to bed – the time at which you go from the living room to the bedroom. Remember, you have only got so much sleep to play with, so you can work out your threshold time by subtracting your average total sleep time from your rising time. Figure 17 will help you select the best threshold and rising time for you.

The time between your threshold time and your rising time is your sleep window – the window of opportunity for you to sleep.

Let's take an example to show how this works. If you estimate that you're sleeping 5½ hours, then you could have a rising time of 7 a.m., and your threshold time to go to bed would be 1.30 a.m. You are free to adjust in either direction from that (have a look at the chart). So you might instead set a rising time of 6.15 a.m., and that would make your threshold time 12.45 a.m. The point is you have set a very tight sleep window, seven nights per week. Write your preferred threshold time below:

My threshold time will be ————

Important note – if you estimate your sleep time as less than 5 hours, it's best for you to use a minimum 5 hours as your sleep window and, if you've been feeling depressed, or are prone to having 'highs', then it's best that you try a minimum of 6 hours.

Changing your sleep window

So what is going to happen if you follow this schedule? Your sleep efficiency will climb rapidly towards 90 per cent. You'll have greatly reduced the amount of time you spend in bed, and that'll force the sleep you do get into the narrow sleep window of opportunity. You'll have increased the proportion of time in bed that you actually sleep. This will make your sleep much more refreshing and uninterrupted. Then, once this has worked, it may be possible for you to stretch the sleep window and get a little bit more sleep. You can track your progress over several weeks in your sleep diary (see page 30–1).

Time to bed

Time to rise	10.30	11.00	11.30	12.00	12.30	1.00	1.30	2.00	2.30	3.00
8.30	10	9.5	9	8.5	8	7.5	7	6.5	6	5.5
8.00	9.5	9	8.5	8	7.5	7	6.5	6	5.5	5
7.30	9	8.5	8	7.5	7	6.5	6	5.5	5	
7.00	8.5	8	7.5	7	6.5	6	5.5	5.5		
6.30	8	7.5	7	6.5	6	5.5	5			
6.00	7.5	7	6.5	6	5.5	5				
5.30	7	6.5	6	5.5	5					
5.00	6.5	6	5.5	5						

Sleep window options

FIGURE 17

So here's the adjustment rule:

> At the end of each week, recalculate your sleep
> efficiency using the sleep efficiency equation
> in Chapter 4 (Figure 9). If it's improving, re-
> ward yourself with an extra 15 minutes in bed
> for the subsequent week.

To use the example we started with, if you use the
adjustment rule this would mean that the sleep window would shift from 5½ to 5¾ hours in the second
week, if you have been sleeping well. Again, if you
manage to increase your sleep efficiency towards
90 per cent, in the third week you can make the
sleep window 6 hours, and then 6¼ hours, 6½
hours, and so on. For each adjustment, you can decide when to set the threshold and getting-up times.

It may take several weeks to increase your total
sleep, but if you do it gradually it can increase without causing your sleep pattern to break up again.

Monitoring your sleep

This can be challenging, so it's worth remembering
the importance of tracking the goals that you set,
and tracking your sleep efficiency. Your diary is
your best friend here because, however you might
feel, the information there gives you an accurate
record of your progress.

9

Dealing with a Racing Mind

Most people with insomnia feel physically tired, even exhausted, but mentally alert. They complain of a racing mind. So let's look at some things we can do to deal with the type of thoughts that are associated with sleeplessness.

Putting the day to rest

We looked at good evening preparations earlier, but we only thought about your activities. Now it's time to think about putting the day to rest. Often, the things that keep us awake are our thoughts, especially going over what happened during the day and thinking ahead to the next day. This isn't a bad thing to do, but it could easily be done in the evening, rather than in bed! Figure 18 contains some suggestions about how you might put the day to rest.

FIGURE 18

1. Set aside 20 minutes in the early evening, the same time every night if possible (say around 7 p.m.).

2. Sit down somewhere you are not going to be disturbed.

3. All you need is a notebook, your diary, and a pen or a computer or other device you can take notes on.

4. Think of what has happened during the day, how events have gone, and how you feel about the kind of day it has been.

5. Write down some of the main points. Put them to rest by committing them to paper. Write down what you feel good about and also what has troubled you. Write down anything you feel you need to do on a 'to do' list, with steps that you can take to tie up any 'loose ends' or 'unfinished business'.

6. Now think about tomorrow and what's coming up. Consider things you are looking forward to as well as things that may cause you worry.

7. Write down your schedule in your diary, or check it if it's already there.

8. Write down anything you are unsure about and make a note in your diary of a time in

the morning when you are going to find
out about it.

9. Try to use your 20 minutes to leave you
feeling more in control. Close the book on
the day.

10. When it comes to bedtime, if these things
come into your mind, remind yourself that
you have already dealt with all of them.

11. If new thoughts come up in bed, note them
down on a piece of paper at your bedside
to be dealt with the following morning.

Accurate thinking

Sometimes, thoughts trouble us because they make
us feel bad. For example, someone with insomnia
might commonly think, 'I am never going to get to
sleep tonight.' This might make them feel worried,
and then they might go on to think that 'I am not
going to be able to cope tomorrow.' This is a vicious
cycle because this could make them feel down, and
then they might have more negative thoughts. A
solution to this kind of thinking is to have a close
look at it – that is, to consider how accurate it is as
a thought process. Let's take that example and use
it in Figure 19. This table is what we might call a
thought evaluator – where we work out whether
the thought is really true or accurate or not.

FIGURE 19

My thoughts about sleep and sleeplessness	How this makes me feel	A more accurate version of my thoughts would be . . .	How this version makes me feel
'It seems as if I am awake half the night and everyone else is sleeping.'	Anxious, annoyed, lonely, jealous	'I probably sleep around 6 hours and have 2 hours awake in bed; that's 75% (three-quarters) not 50%. Also if there are 1 million people living in this city and half of them are adults, maybe 50,000 are having serious problems. Everyone else is not sleeping!'	Reassured, more optimistic, less angry

'I'm never going to get to sleep tonight.'	Demoralised, out of control	'Almost certainly I will fall asleep. I always get some sleep. The average in my diary was 6 hours and I never got less than 3–4 hours.'	More accepting, relieved, more relaxed
'I'm so tired I just can't concentrate. It's because I slept so badly last night.'	Hopeless, pre-occupied with sleep, irritable	'My concentration is not just down to my sleep. I've slept worse than I did last night and felt better during the day. Maybe I'm bored, or doing too much at once, or ...'	More in control, able to focus

So the challenge is to have the courage to work out whether your thoughts really are accurate. If you can correct your thinking in this way, it will be much less threatening and demoralising. Use a version of this table in a notebook or on a computer or phone to work out your own negative thoughts and replace them with more accurate and less alarming ones!

Stop trying to sleep

This is so important. As soon as you start giving your attention to sleeplessness, it'll take over your thinking and will lead to you *trying* to fall asleep. One remedy is to have a more accepting approach to your wakefulness. In other words, the problem is not so much being awake – the problem is your emotional response to being awake. If you can correct that, you will feel a whole lot better – and be more likely to get back to sleep.

Your problem is not so much being awake but having a strong emotional response to being awake

During the night, when there's nothing else to do, our thinking can become very troublesome, so another approach is to stop trying so hard to sleep by using our sense of humour to address the problem directly. Below is a transcript of a conversation between a patient and their therapist which demonstrates that sometimes we think too much and get things out of proportion.

Hopefully, these different pieces of advice about giving up trying will be helpful. Remember the thin line – your focus should be on following the Cognitive Behavioural Therapy programme and not so much on your sleep itself.

FIGURE 20

The Use of Humour in Paradoxical Intention Therapy

Patient: It is pretty awful really when I think about it. I can't sleep at night, and then, to make matters worse, insomnia just ruins my day.

Therapist: What do you mean?

Patient: Well, I can't think straight, and I get irritable, and I don't get through as much work as I should.

Therapist:	That's shocking.
Patient:	What's shocking?
Therapist:	Well, that you don't get through your work. I mean, that's pretty bad.
Patient:	Well, it's not that I don't get my work done, it's more that . . .
Therapist:	Sorry, you are the one that said you didn't get through your work. So what effect does that have?
Patient:	Well, it might get noticed. I mean my boss might notice it.
Therapist:	Really! . . . I guess he wouldn't like that?
Patient:	Erm, no, he'd probably have something to say about it. It could affect my job.
Therapist:	Wow, that's worrying. You're not getting through your work, your boss is maybe going to notice, and you might lose your job.
Patient:	Yeah. It's possible.

Therapist:	Have you thought about reducing your financial commitments?
Patient:	What?
Therapist:	. . . like maybe giving up your golf club membership, or taking the kids out of private school?
Patient:	No, no, I haven't, but why . . . ?
Therapist:	I mean, if these things are likely to happen then it would be best to take responsible action.
Patient:	I think this is maybe getting a bit exaggerated, I mean, it's not that bad . . . it's not even likely, I don't think.
Therapist:	Thank goodness for that! (Takes out handkerchief and mops brow).
Patient:	(Smiles)
Therapist:	(Smiles, laughs) I thought I was going to have an anxiety attack there!
Patient:	(Laughs) Yeah, I'm like a dog with a bone about this sleep problem!
Therapist:	I was just about to check if I had some loose change to give you!!

Patient:	(Laughs) . . . very thoughtful of you.
Therapist:	You know, I think you're just worrying too hard in every department . . . about sleep . . . and also during the day. Why don't you give yourself a break?
Patient:	(Laughs) You're not the first person to have suggested that!

10

Evaluating How You Feel During the Day

Use the thought evaluator to deal with your daytime thinking too

At the beginning of this book we talked about how insomnia is a 24-hour problem. It's important to improve how you feel during the day, as well as how you feel at night. So when you're using the thought evaluator in the last chapter (Figure 19), also use it for the thoughts that you have during the day. For example, it might occur to you that you are feeling extremely tired and 'That's because of my poor sleep last night', but think about whether there are any other explanations for you feeling tired right now. Perhaps you're overdoing it and need a rest. Likewise, you might have made a bad job of something. It could be all too easy to blame your sleep for that, but maybe you've just made a bad job of it! You have to weigh up how much poor sleep adds to your daytime difficulties, and to what extent the difficulties would be there anyway. So you should be working on solutions by improving your sleep, and also by improving how you cope in the daytime.

11

Making Lasting Improvements to Your Sleep

As we draw to a close, we should talk about how to make improvements last. There are three headlines here:

1. Use all the CBT advice: try not to pick and choose.

2. Recognise that it takes time and that it may be tough to make lasting changes.

3. Deal positively with any setbacks.

Keeping it all together

While there's a lot of tightly packed information in this book, try to avoid the temptation of treating it like a menu. In other words, it is not really meant for dipping into and selecting items that appeal to you.

If some parts are completely irrelevant to you, because you simply don't have a problem in that area, then fair enough; otherwise, complete every bit you can if you want to make your sleep better in the long term.

It's going to be tough

It can be tough to overcome insomnia. It really does involve breaking up an old pattern and building a new one, completely changing the way you think about sleep, and believing that you too can become a normal sleeper.

While it will be a challenge, sticking to the programme will bear its own fruits in time. You need to be tolerant with yourself if, at times, you feel that you're failing, and you need to encourage yourself to get back on track. Elements such as the new sleep window and the quarter of an hour rule are the most difficult bits for people to carry out. But they're also among the best strategies. Staying motivated is the key to making a lasting improvement to your sleep.

Dealing with setbacks

There are two ways you might experience a setback. You might be able to create a new sleep pattern for a while but then feel like giving up because it is hard work to keep going. This is perfectly normal and to be expected. It's part of human nature; so don't be discouraged. The second thing is that, even once your sleep pattern is back to normal, you'll have a bad night or a period of poor sleep. The difference between you and the good sleeper at these times is simply that the good sleeper doesn't think that they're developing insomnia. You've had it before, so a change of thinking is definitely required here too – don't panic, just go back and work your way through the methods outlined in this book for a while.

Good luck as you try to overcome your insomnia!

Other Things that Might Help

This book provides you with an introduction to insomnia and what you can do to overcome it. You may find this is all that you need to achieve a big improvement. On the other hand, you may feel that you need more information and help, and in that case there are some longer, more detailed self-help books available. You could ask your GP if there is a 'Books on Prescription' scheme running in your area. The following books are recommended.

Overcoming Insomnia and Sleep Problems by Colin A. Espie, published by Robinson. This includes a script that you can record to create your own relaxation CD.

The Insomnia Answer by Paul Glovinsky and Art Spielman, published by Penguin.

Sometimes the self-help approach works better if you have someone supporting you. Ask your GP if there is anyone at the surgery who would be able to work through your self-help book with you. Some surgeries have IAPT (Improving Access to Psychological Therapies) workers who would be able to help in this way, or who might offer general support. He or she is likely to be able to spend more time with you than your GP, and may be able to offer follow-up appointments.

For some people, a self-help approach may not be enough. If this is the case for you, don't despair – there are other kinds of help available.

Talk to your GP – make an appointment to talk through the different treatment options on offer to you. Your GP can refer you to an NHS therapist for Cognitive Behavioural Therapy. Most places now have CBT available on the NHS, although there can be a considerable waiting list. Don't be put off if you've not found working through a CBT-based self-help manual right for you – talking to a therapist can make a big difference. If an NHS therapist isn't available in your area, or you would prefer not to wait to see one, ask your GP to recommend a private therapist or a local sleep centre, which may have specialised expertise.

Although CBT is widely recommended for insomnia problems, there are other kinds of therapy available which you could also discuss with your GP.

Medication can be helpful for some people, particularly in the short term, and sometimes a combination of medication and psychological therapy can be appropriate. You need to discuss this form of treatment and any possible side-effects with your GP to work out whether it is right for you.

The following organisations offer help and advice on sleep problems, and you may find them a useful source of information:

British Sleep Society

Provides useful information about sleep and sleep disorders and contact details for sleep centres and specialists.

Website: www.sleeping.org.uk
Email: admin@sleepsociety.org.uk

Sleepio

Provides online assessment and treatment services. Also has a free relaxation MP3 to download.

Website: www.sleepio.com
Email: hello@sleepio.com

Mind

The leading mental-health charity in England and Wales.

Website: www.mind.org.uk
Tel: 020 8519 2122

Mental Health Foundation

The Mental Health Foundation has a free download guide entitled *How too… Sleep better* on their website (printed copy also on sale).

Website: www.mentalhealth.org.uk

British Association for Behavioural and Cognitive Psychotherapies (BABCP)

Provides contact details for therapists in your area, both NHS and private.

Website: www.babcp.org.uk
Email: babcp@babcp.com
Tel: 0161 705 4304

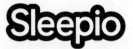

Sleepio

Need more help with your sleep? Try Sleepio – the online sleep improvement programme developed by Prof. Colin A. Espie.

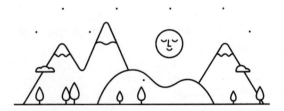